FERONIA

THE LITTLE GIRL WHO LEARNED TO FLY FREE

Nola Anne Hennessy

This book may be ordered through booksellers, purchased directly from the publisher at www.serenidadconsulting.com/buy-our-books, and also by contacting the publisher directly at:

Serenidad Consulting Pty Ltd
PO Box 881
Sanctuary Cove QLD 4212
Australia

Email: enquiry@serenidadconsulting.com
www.serenidadconsulting.com/contact-us/

ISBN: 978-0-9874599-9-2 (sc)
ISBN: 978-0-0993951-0-8 (e)

Australian National Library CIP

This book is written in such as way as to appeal to and assist children who have experienced trauma at an early age. The storyline is based on similar experiences of the author, downplayed or altered where necessary to enable ease of reading and comprehension by children under the age of 15.

The author does not dispense medical advice or prescribe the use of any technique as a form of treatment for a physical, emotional or mental condition. In the event you use any of the information in this book to assist yourself or another person, which is your constitutional and/or legal right, the author and the publisher assume no responsibility for your choices and actions.

Cover Design by: the Author

Published by: Serenidad Consulting Pty Ltd, 1/1/2017

DEDICATION

This book is dedicated to my father, Robert Alexander Hennessy, who shared unselfishly, shone and laughed brightly, and remained loyal to me all his life and at his death.

Feronia – The Little Girl Who Learned To Fly Free

CHAPTER 1

Feronia learned to forgive others at a very young age. Even the ones who'd hurt her the most.

She was challenged from the very beginning of life, and learned to navigate a rough path where people were sometimes very bad to her. But, she remained determined to be kind and compassionate no matter what.

For all of her life, from when she was a little girl, Feronia loved to dance, sing, write, read, and play outside in nature as often as she was allowed. She lived in an old weatherboard house in a very large and bustling city, with her mother and a sibling she didn't like very much. Her daddy had left just before she was born. Feronia only saw her daddy a few times until she was in Kindergarten, then the visits together stopped for nearly 20 years.

Feronia's mother was as tough as an old, sun-baked leather boot but she probably wasn't born a nasty person; at least Feronia didn't think so. What seemed obvious to Feronia throughout her childhood and later in life, was that because her mother's life had not gone the way her mother expected it to, she took out her anger and pain, and blaming, on Feronia.

Her mother always spoke abruptly and forcefully to her and regularly left handprint marks on Feronia's legs whenever things got too much for her to cope with. And, of course, Feronia's sibling learned how to treat people, by watching what their mother did and said. That made Feronia's life with them really challenging, at times utterly miserable, and very hard for her to manage in isolation from her school friends and grandparents.

Divide and conquer seemed to be her mother's motto and isolating her from her best friend Sally was the ultimate manipulation and control technique. Feronia was always blamed for what went wrong in the house, at work, at school and in life. She was frequently hurt, in all sorts of ways including with words, and these experiences not only left some bruises on the outside, they created scars on the inside that no-one could see. The outer bruises would heal, eventually, but the inner ones were much harder for her to fix, especially while she was so young.

Feronia was the youngest and by far the happiest member of her immediate family however, as a result of being so bubbly and playful, she became the target for all those people around her who lived unsatisfying and unhappy lives.

She was the second and also unwanted child borne of a marriage that was angry, sharp and cold. Feronia's mother was always a victim of something, always complaining and Feronia found it hard to navigate the negative stream of talk that always filled the air in her home. It felt to her like she was dodging flying arrows every day.

But the good news was, this meant that every time Feronia went to visit her only grandparents, who lived far away in a pretty seaside town, that's when she felt totally safe, happy and loved unconditionally.

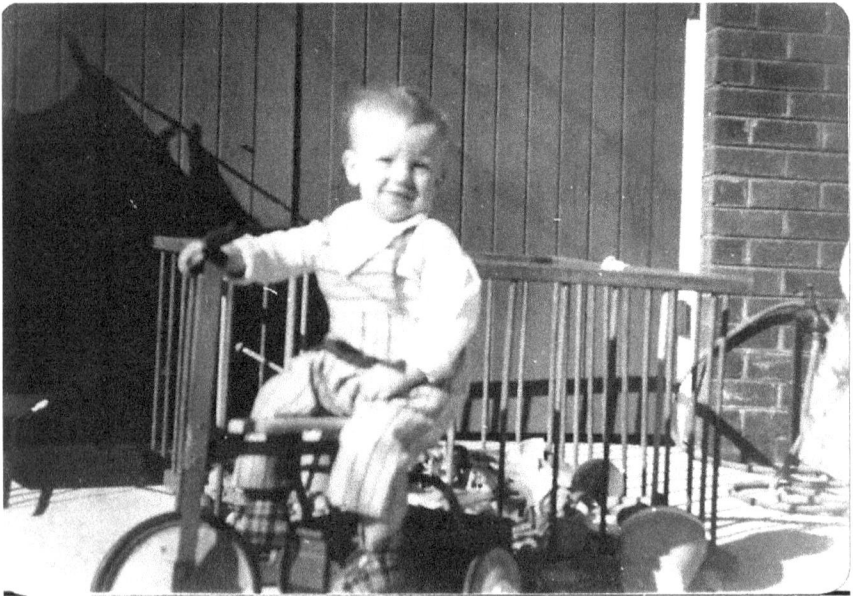

Feronia's grandparents nurtured her in the same way that Feronia later nurtured her own child. Feronia learned the right value system from her grandparents, how to really care for people and things, even when life didn't always go as planned.

Even now, as a middle aged woman, Feronia continues to nurture important relationships in her life and also the gardens that surround her homes – with nourishment, gentleness, love and good support.

CHAPTER 2

When Feronia was about seven her mother met a man who had a big, hairy wart on his left cheek. He smelled sickly sweet like he'd been rolled in candy and radiated a falseness and pretentious charm. He always put out waves of affection and compliments that were too warm and nice. And, his brow and the palms of his hands were always sweaty.

All that, mixed with his hairy hands and the tufts of black hair that would come out from the top of his shirts, even from behind his tightly knotted tie, his appearance made Feronia wince and withdraw from him at the first chance possible each time he visited.

It was plain to see that Feronia's mother liked him a lot and he was always at Feronia's house watching Feronia while she did things, reaching out to touch her and pulling her close to his body. Feronia didn't like what he did or said, but because she was frightened of her mother, and careful so as not to say something that could set her mother off into an angry rant, Feronia said nothing about his behavior for many months.

Feronia felt very uncomfortable and wary whenever he was around at their house. Many times he would squeeze her body in a way that felt wrong to Feronia. But she was still too young to understand the gravity of what was going on and why he was behaving this way.

Quite to her surprise one day, when she felt she'd finally had enough of her life in that home, Feronia packed her little pink and white carry purse with all the special things she thought she'd need on her journey to freedom, the first stop being her grandparent's house.

Feronia put in her purse a change of underwear, a hankie (like her Grandma always said she must do when she went out anywhere), socks, bath soap, and a comb for her hair. Feronia was not allowed to have long, flowing hair, so she was able to fix her hair herself most of the time. It was quick to comb straight when she was being hurried along.

On the cold, misty winter's morning that Feronia decided to run away from home, her mother heard her open the squeaky front door of the house and saw her running to the side gate. She ran after Feronia and stopped her from leaving by grabbing her arm and pulling her backwards, so hard that Feronia spun in a circle. Feronia quickly told her mother that she was leaving to get away from her mother's horrible boyfriend, and why. Well, that was the reason she was willing to share; the one she thought would make the most sense to her mother.

Feronia's mother got very cross with her, wacked her hard on her back between her shoulders, dragged her by the arm into the house, and locked her in her bedroom. Feronia sobbed for the rest of the day and when she finally got let out of the shared, unheated and bitterly cold bedroom, she told her mother again that the man who visited them wasn't being good.

She also warned her mother that if the man was going to come and live with them, then she would leave and never come back. Feronia meant it, but Feronia's mother didn't seem to want to understand why or care much for how upset Feronia was.

Running away from home, and getting away from that bad situation, was Feronia's only choice in order for her to take control of her life.

At the time she didn't know it as that, a choice, but later in her life when similar upsetting things would happen, she always remembered that first time when she found the courage to act; when she decided it was time for her to be free from all the negatives. Feronia so longed to be surrounded by happiness and peace, not anger and cruelty.

The more her mother and sibling, and others around her, were unfriendly or nasty or cruel towards her, the more Feronia worked hard to be a friendly, fun, playful people-person. All the denials, the accusations, the criticisms, the beatings and other cruelties simply made Feronia more determined to be nice to people, even the ones who hurt her the most.

She knew that while she was stuck in that house, she had to make the most of a bad situation.

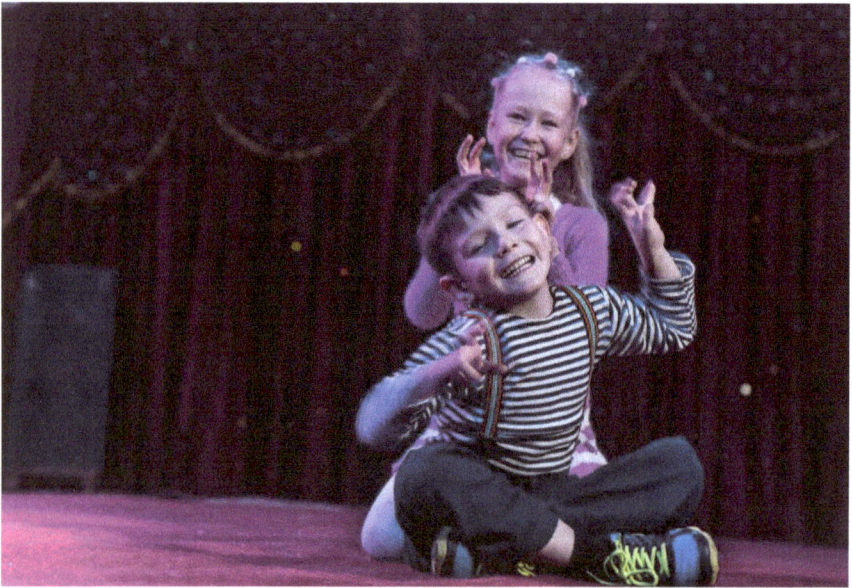

CHAPTER 3

Despite the negative way that members of her family and others treated her, how Feronia managed her own feelings was a true reflection of her bold, courageous spirit, and her playful, happy and positive nature.

To maintain a positive view of life, Feronia would dance and sing, read, play in the garden, write plays and then get the neighbourhood's children to come around and act out the many characters there were to play. She stayed active, focused on happy things, and true to her nature.

When Feronia was still primary school age she found a way to get to the large, cream-bricked church that was only a few streets uphill from where she lived. She was invited to attend the church's Sunday School class and, on the occasions when her mother let her go, she really loved the companionship of the other children.

At that time, and forever in the future, being in church always helped her to feel safe and cared about. Feronia started to develop an understanding of God back then.

As a grown woman, nearly four decades later in her life, she was fortunate to experience a very special, spiritual connection with God again. It's this later connection and gaining a very high awareness of who she is inside, that have brought her much inner peace and an even greater understanding of everything and everyone around her.

As a young, primary school-age child Feronia was very self-reliant and also most reliable. Her mother depended on her to do household chores while she was at work.

Once Feronia turned 10 she was allocated the bulk of the chores to do around the house, which resulted in her getting very dirty, wet, tired or blistered.

Feronia also worked hard at her primary school, to please the teachers and principal. She was happy within her circle of friends and there was a routine about school. Even so, by comparison to most it was a very strict and regimented school where boys and girls marched everywhere, including into class, and wore heavy starched uniforms.

The standard of education was considered high, but the atmosphere at the school lacked something. In later years Feronia came to realize it lacked empathy. It was high on discipline and low on compassion.

Being so resourceful, Feronia was always active helping out others. She learned to do more than most children her age and, in reality, this was a habit she formed in order to please her mother and keep her from ranting and raving about "achieving", which her mother did incessantly.

On most days Feronia felt that she was managing her emotions and responses to people as best she could. At times though, she could feel her heartbeat rushing and her body would feel really tight and congested on the inside. She didn't know why, but she felt like she was suffocating inside her own body and couldn't get out.

Other times she'd vary from feeling very cautious and wary, to being totally overwhelmed with fear whenever she was alone with her mother, sibling, the mother's boyfriend or one of Feronia's uncles whom they used to see a lot.

In fact, anyone who reminded her of any one of these people, even if she just saw them at a distance in the street, would set off these feelings and body sensations inside Feronia.

Feronia seemed to develop eyes in the back of her head, because she actually became quite good at sensing people approaching from behind.

When Feronia was most upset, she used laughter or tears to release pain and frustration, and she would also take time out to be on her own whenever she found people around her being cruel and nasty, or sleazy like the hairy boyfriend and her uncle.

Unfortunately, she used to have nightmares whenever she slept, even during the daytime when she took a nap sometimes.

Feronia didn't realize at that time, when she was so little, that she had suffered lots of different kinds of trauma and that the responses and sensations she felt were actually her body and spirit giving her loud signals that she needed time to heal from all the times she'd been hurt.

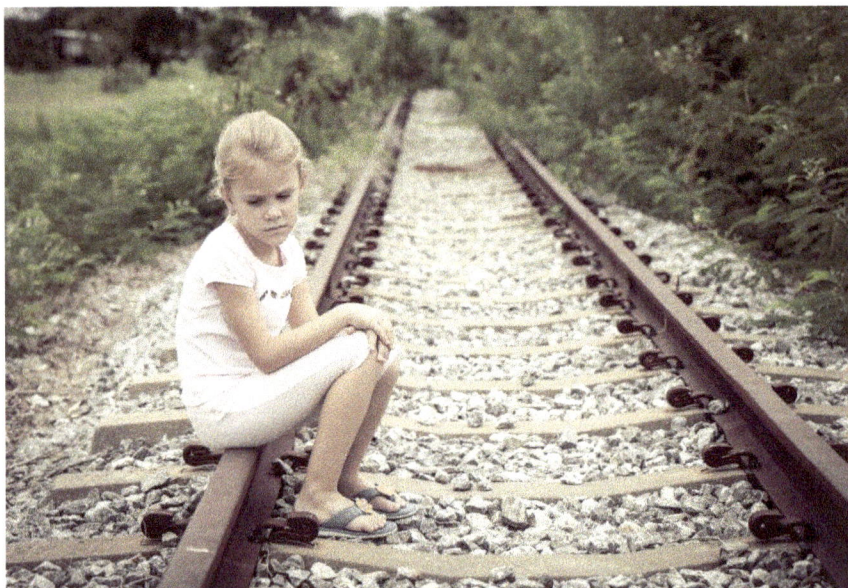

CHAPTER 4

Feronia always knew her uncle, and other bad men in her life at that time, were being sinful with their words and eyes but, in her family, children were always told never to speak back to an adult, and to "be seen and not heard".

Her grandparents had made this rule back when they first had children, but Feronia soon figured that maybe they hadn't taught their own four children how to apply the rule in all different circumstances. Feronia's mother had certainly learned the rule word-for-word, but not how to balance rules with reality. She also didn't know how to serve rules up on a plate, alongside a generous portion of love and compassion.

What Feronia saw early on was a strong imbalance in how relationship rules were applied. Where her mother sided with applying rules without compromise and dishing out punishments "just because", with the majority of these punishments dished out to Feronia, there was rarely any recognition given to the good things that were done.

In God's eyes, relationship rules are founded on truth, honor, faithfulness, honesty, gentleness and kindness.

Feronia knew that no-one is perfect and that everyone makes mistakes. She was only starting to understand the principle that 'what goes around, comes around'.

What she couldn't see so clearly as a child she learned later in life as an adult - that when people do bad deeds, their judgment day will eventually come.

God sees and hears all, and whilst we can forget or ignore some things ourselves, God knows full well everything that has gone before - who lied and who was honest, who did the hurting and who was hurt, who was harsh and who was kind, who helped and who sat back doing nothing.

That's the wonderful thing about trusting in universal justice, rather than taking justice into your own hands. Even though her life was not the best, Feronia didn't ever take revenge. She always thought the best approach was to extract herself from the bad places and people, and let them come unstuck on their own. She always knew the universe would take care of punishing bad people, one way or the other.

Even though, as a child, she didn't know God's true wisdom, as she'd rarely been allowed to go to Sunday School or learn much about spirituality, she was in fact living that divine value system without even knowing it.

And each time she didn't take revenge, it was like she gained more strength to stay strong in amongst all the cruelty and badness that was around her.

For Feronia, not being allowed or encouraged to speak up seemed completely at odds with real justice. She knew instinctively that the sad part about not encouraging a child to speak up and contribute to conversations, was that they then learned not to stand up for themselves at all; not to speak up in their own defence when it was most important.

It was quite a few years and a move into middle school, before Feronia had the opportunity to take more control of her own outcomes. When she did make those moves a whole new world of fun, freedom, and empowerment opened up for her. It was like the universe was waiting for the right set of circumstances to be placed in Feronia's path, for her to then have the right choices to make. And Feronia sure did make lots of the right choices when the time came.

CHAPTER 5

Because Feronia's mother didn't seem to have much money and good, nourishing food was pretty scarce on their dinner table, Feronia used her experience in keeping house and cleaning when she was little, to win herself a number of after school jobs starting when she turned 12. Her very first paid job working for a large supermarket chain as a packer of groceries, was also the first time she actually paid income tax to the government.

This was a major turning point for Feronia and she felt like she was contributing in a big way to the wider world that surrounded her. She felt like she was really growing up and had the chance to make something of herself, in the way she wanted.

By the time she turned 15 Feronia was an experienced supervisor of others, and by age 16 she was a senior manager working long, part-time hours for a very busy tourist industry business, as well as completing her last 18 months of high school and working towards her acceptance into university.

Feronia kept herself busy all the time, was out and about with other people, some very nice people, and this was a major contributor to her healing from the damage that had been done in her younger years.

The more nice people she encountered and interacted with, the more she was able to see that not all people have bad intentions or do bad things. She needed that reassurance and found it.

Another contributor to her healing and sense of wellness was the time she spent with her grandparents helping with community activities as a volunteer. Volunteering became Feronia's lifeline to grateful and happy people, from as early as 10 years of age when she would help her grandparents with their community and charity work.

As the visits to her grandparents became a little less frequent while she went through middle and high school, Feronia made choices to engage with people, away from her own home surroundings, at every opportunity. She became a tutor of young primary age children, helped out on committees and working groups in her middle and high schools, and would babysit smaller children at every opportunity.

During her middle and high school years Feronia did make a lot of mistakes and learned several valuable lessons, but the most marked thing that changed was her mother and sibling were not around at home as much. The dynamic of the family was pretty much still the same, but their absence meant that Feronia had more time to heal in between episodes. Time became Feronia's real healer.

Later in life she went on to teach other people the value of taking time with important decisions and actions, especially the ones that have an impact on your health and wellbeing.

Feronia did experience working for some quite sleazy men during her middle and high school years, however their impact on her and power to change her life's course was greatly diminished by the time she finished high school.

Feronia had come to realize her own inner strength, had healed from the nightmares and no longer had fear responses when she saw the people who had hurt, and were still hurting, her. It seemed to her that she was being given these bad events to teach her lots of things. And in so many respects, Feronia remained eager to learn.

By the time Feronia finished high school at age 17, she had matured so much that people thought she was years older than she actually was. Feronia had the air and confidence of one much older, a manner that spoke of wisdom beyond her years, and a positive attitude that saw no boundaries.

She knew full well that bad people would still do bad things, and maybe never get caught out by authorities. She also knew that good people get set up and blamed for bad things that happen, when it was never their fault in the first place.

By age 17 Feronia was so experienced in the workplace and in life, she only had one future in mind – a future that allowed for freedom from the emotional and mental chains her mother still laid around her, and a future that would enable her to live out her dreams and wishes, without relying on other people to make it happen for her.

Everything in Feronia's life thus far, had spelled a path for her that was all about empowerment, strength, integrity, honesty and doing good for others. Her own life had taught her so many lessons and she was always the first to speak up in other people's defence, but most times she found her passionate words fell on deaf ears. She wanted to help fix these injustices.

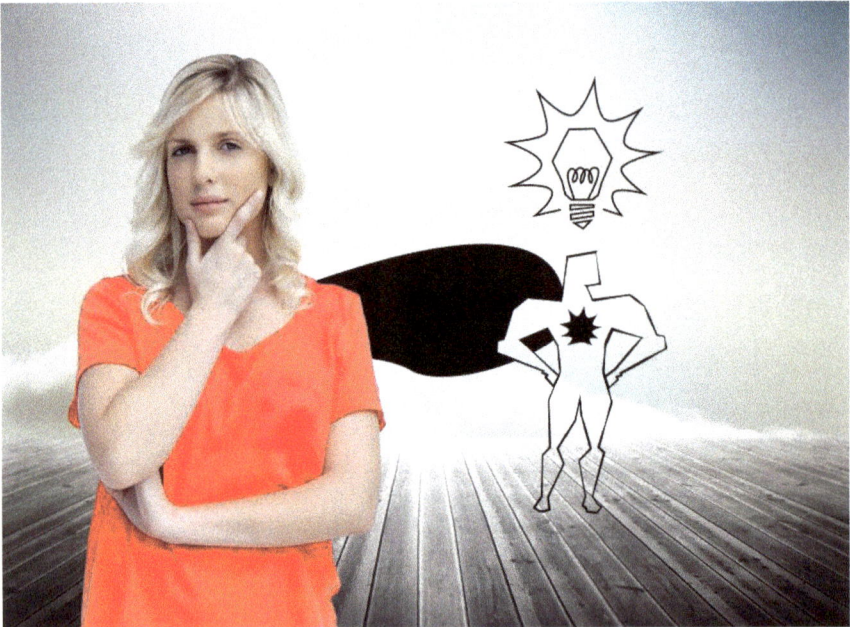

CHAPTER 6

Feronia's journey to freedom had well and truly begun by age 17.

With all her experience in the workplace, and with two years of solid training under her belt, she was elevated to a very senior position as the second-in-charge manager, running an international hotel in the country's capital city. She was only 19 years old, not even legally an adult, but she had already reached a senior leadership position.

Feronia hadn't planned for that to happen, it just did, and often when she's looked back on those early career years she realizes that it was her strong people and planning skills that got her there. She was really well organized, and that meant she just got things done without hassle and fuss.

Often times she was exhausted working night shifts and managing people who were always much older than her. Those days and nights, being in charge when the General Manager was home with his own family and having time off, was a crucial time for Feronia to learn even more about ethics and integrity. She did make some mistakes but she also got to experience things that many people never have the chance or inclination to experience.

Meeting and dining with celebrities, officials and other VIPs were normal activities for her. Planning and managing the budgets, the rosters, the timetables of events, and making sure that staff did the right thing and guests behaved themselves, made for a busy life. And all the while, she studied hard to pass her tests and exams at college.

By the time she turned 21, and officially became an adult with the right to vote, Feronia had embedded herself in her second career. She had the full attention and interest of some of the world's most powerful and well-known people.

This time in her life marked the beginning of a second and most exciting chapter for her. This was when she knew that the traumas of her childhood were passed, her healing had happened and, whilst some of the inner scars were still there, she ignored those and chose to carry forward the lessons instead.

And, as Feronia's life continued to change and she grew in her career, fell in love at 23 and even travelled to the other side of the world to begin a new life, the memories of her grandparents remained with her.

She never told her grandparents all the bad things that had happened to her over those years but she sensed that her grandparents knew more than was spoken about.

Still now, long after her grandparents have passed away, Feronia remains grateful for the private peaceful sanctuary they gave her. They created her first safe place, and she knew deep inside that feeling safe was critical to being able to heal. Feronia knew that when she felt safe, she was empowered to grow her self-awareness and resilience.

For all the bad experiences of her childhood, Feronia had come out of it well-adjusted and powerful. Her childhood was moulding her into the successful, celebrated woman she would become, and she didn't even know it.

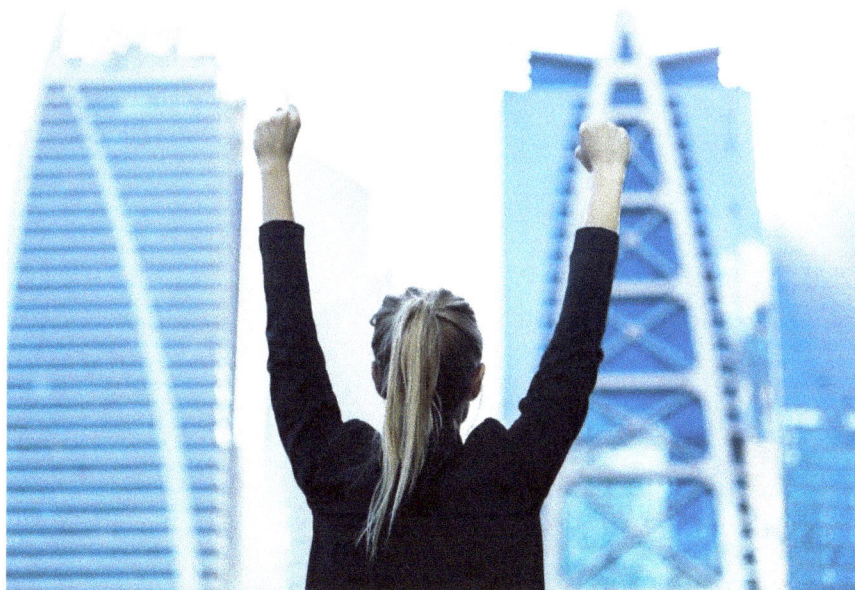

www.ingramcontent.com/pod-product-compliance
Lightning Source LLC
Chambersburg PA
CBHW041302040426

42334CB00028BA/3127